CONTENTS

INTRODUCTION

Definition and Explanation of the Alkaline Diet

The alkaline diet, also known as the alkaline ash diet or acid-alkaline diet, is based on the idea that certain foods can affect the acidity or alkalinity (pH) levels in our body. Proponents of this diet claim that consuming alkaline foods can help maintain optimal health by balancing the body's pH levels.

The pH Scale

To understand the alkaline diet, it's important to have a basic understanding of the pH scale. The pH scale ranges from 0 to 14, with 7 being neutral. Values below 7 indicate acidity, while values above 7 indicate alkalinity. Our bodies naturally maintain a slightly alkaline pH level, typically around 7.4.

Acid-Forming and Alkaline-Forming Foods

According to the alkaline diet, foods can be categorized as either acid-forming or alkaline-forming based on the effect they have on the body's pH levels. Acid-forming foods, such as meat, dairy, refined grains, and processed foods, are believed to increase acidity in the body. On the other hand, alkaline-forming foods, including fruits, vegetables, nuts, and legumes, are thought to have an alkalizing effect.

Acid-Base Balance

Advocates of the alkaline diet claim that maintaining a slightly alkaline pH level can have numerous health benefits. They argue that excess acidity in the body can lead to various health problems, such as inflammation, osteoporosis, and impaired immune function. By consuming a predominantly alkaline diet, they believe you can restore the acid-base balance and improve overall health.

Potential Benefits of Following an Alkaline Diet

While the alkaline diet has gained popularity in recent years, it's important to note that scientific evidence supporting its benefits is limited. However, proponents suggest several potential advantages of following this diet:

1. Improved Digestion: The alkaline diet encourages the consumption of fruits and vegetables, which are rich in fiber. A high-fiber diet can promote healthy digestion, prevent constipation, and support gut health.

2. Increased Fruit and Vegetable Intake: Following an alkaline diet often leads to a higher intake of fruits and vegetables, which are packed with essential vitamins, minerals, and antioxidants. These nutrients play a vital role in overall health and can help reduce the risk of chronic diseases.

3. Weight Management: The alkaline diet promotes whole, unprocessed foods and discourages the consumption of refined sugars and saturated fats. This approach, combined with a focus on plant-based foods, can contribute to weight management and support a healthy body weight.

4. Potential Anti-Inflammatory Effects: Some alkaline-forming foods, such as leafy greens and certain fruits, are known for their anti-inflammatory properties. By consuming these foods, individuals may experience a reduction in inflammation and related health issues.

CHAPTER ONE

Understanding pH and

Acid-Alkaline Balance

Explanation of pH Scale and Its Relevance to Health

The pH scale is a measurement system used to determine the acidity or alkalinity of a substance. It measures the concentration of hydrogen ions in a solution, ranging from 0 to 14. A pH value of 7 is considered neutral, while values below 7 indicate acidity, and values above 7 indicate alkalinity. In the context of health, understanding the pH scale and its relevance is crucial to maintaining a balanced and optimal internal environment within the body.

Acidic and Alkaline Substances

To comprehend the pH scale's significance, it is essential to distinguish between acidic and alkaline substances. Acids are substances that release hydrogen ions when dissolved in water, leading to an increase in the concentration of positively charged hydrogen ions (H+). Examples of acidic substances include lemon juice and vinegar. On the other hand, alkaline substances, also known as bases, decrease the concentration of hydrogen ions and have a higher concentration of hydroxide ions (OH-). Baking soda and soap are examples of alkaline substances.

The pH Scale and Health

The human body has different pH levels in various areas and fluids. Blood, for instance, has a slightly alkaline pH ranging from 7.35 to 7.45. The pH levels in other parts of the body, such as the stomach, skin, and urine, vary to perform specific functions effectively.

Maintaining the body's pH balance is crucial for overall health. The body has intricate mechanisms to regulate pH levels and keep them within the appropriate range. Various organs and systems work together to maintain this balance, including the kidneys, lungs, and buffers present in bodily fluids.

Acid-Alkaline Balance in the Body

The concept of acid-alkaline balance refers to the equilibrium between acidic and alkaline substances in the body. This balance plays a vital role in supporting optimal cellular function and overall health. The body works hard to keep the blood pH within a narrow range because even slight deviations can disrupt biochemical processes.

When the body is in a healthy state, it can effectively neutralize excess acid or alkaline substances through buffering systems. Buffers are substances that help stabilize pH levels by accepting or donating hydrogen ions. The most critical buffer system in the body is the bicarbonate-carbonic acid buffer system, which operates in the blood and other bodily fluids.

Effects of pH Imbalance on Overall Health

When the body's acid-alkaline balance is disrupted, it can lead to various health issues. An excessively acidic or alkaline environment can affect enzyme activity, cellular function, and nutrient absorption. Here are some potential effects of pH imbalance on overall health:

1. **Digestive Disturbances:** The stomach has a highly acidic environment (pH around 2) to aid in the digestion of food. Excessive acidity or alkalinity in the stomach can disrupt the proper breakdown of food, leading to indigestion, heartburn, or acid reflux.

2. **Mineral Imbalances:** pH imbalances can affect the body's ability to absorb and utilize minerals effectively. For example, high acidity can contribute to calcium loss from bones, leading to osteoporosis, while alkalosis (excessive alkalinity) can interfere with potassium and magnesium levels.

3. **Impaired Immune Function:** The immune system relies on an optimal pH balance to function efficiently. An overly acidic environment can compromise immune cell activity, making the body more susceptible to infections and diseases.

4. **Inflammation:** Acidic conditions in the body can contribute to chronic inflammation, which is associated with various health conditions, including arthritis, cardiovascular disease, and certain types of cancer. Maintaining a balanced pH can help reduce inflammation and promote better overall health.

5. **Impact on Skin Health:** The pH level of the skin plays a crucial role in maintaining its barrier function and protecting against harmful bacteria and irritants. Disruptions in the skin's pH balance can lead to dryness, irritation, acne breakouts,

and other skin conditions. Using pH-balanced skincare products can help support the skin's natural acid mantle and promote healthier skin.

6. **Energy Levels and Fatigue:** pH imbalances can also affect energy levels and contribute to fatigue. When the body is too acidic, it can hinder cellular energy production and slow down metabolic processes. This can result in feelings of fatigue, sluggishness, and reduced overall vitality.

7. **Dental Health:** The pH balance in the mouth is essential for maintaining good oral health. A pH below 5.5 can contribute to tooth erosion and dental decay, as acids can demineralize tooth enamel. Maintaining a slightly alkaline pH in the mouth through proper oral hygiene and a balanced diet can help protect teeth from acid-related damage.

8. **Digestive Disorders:** pH imbalances can disrupt the delicate ecosystem of the gut microbiome, leading to digestive disorders such as irritable bowel syndrome (IBS) and inflammatory bowel disease (IBD). The gut relies on a slightly acidic environment to support the growth of beneficial bacteria and maintain a healthy balance. pH disruptions can negatively impact gut health and contribute to gastrointestinal issues.

9. **Athletic Performance:** Maintaining an optimal pH balance is crucial for athletes and individuals involved in intense physical activities. Acidosis, which refers to excessive acidity in the body, can impair muscle function, reduce endurance, and delay recovery. By ensuring a proper acid-alkaline

balance, athletes can enhance their performance and minimize the risk of muscle fatigue and injury.

10. **General Well-being:** The overall impact of pH balance on health cannot be overstated. When the body's pH is in balance, it functions optimally, and all physiological processes can occur smoothly. By paying attention to dietary choices, managing stress levels, staying hydrated, and adopting a healthy lifestyle, individuals can support their body's acid-alkaline balance and promote well-being.

CHAPTER TWO

Alkaline Foods and Their Benefits

List and Description of Alkaline Foods

Alkaline foods are those that have an alkalizing effect on the body when consumed. These foods help to balance the pH levels in the body by neutralizing excess acid, which can contribute to various health issues. Including alkaline foods in your diet can promote overall well-being and support optimal health. Here is a list of alkaline foods along with their descriptions:

1. Leafy Green Vegetables:
    - Spinach, kale, Swiss chard, and other leafy greens are highly alkaline and rich in essential nutrients. They are excellent sources of vitamins A, C, and K, as well as folate and minerals like iron and calcium.

2. Cruciferous Vegetables:
    - Vegetables such as broccoli, cauliflower, Brussels sprouts, and cabbage are alkaline-rich and packed with dietary fiber. They also contain powerful

antioxidants and phytochemicals that support detoxification and reduce the risk of chronic diseases.

3. Citrus Fruits:

- Citrus fruits like lemons, limes, and grapefruits, although acidic in nature, have an alkalizing effect on the body. They are abundant in vitamin C, which boosts the immune system and aids in collagen production.

4. Root Vegetables:

- Root vegetables such as sweet potatoes, carrots, beets, and radishes are alkaline-forming and provide a good source of fiber, vitamins, and minerals. They are also known for their antioxidant properties.

5. Nuts and Seeds:

- Almonds, chia seeds, flaxseeds, and pumpkin seeds are alkaline foods that offer a wealth of nutritional benefits. They are rich in healthy fats, protein, fiber, and various essential vitamins and minerals.

6. Herbal Teas:

- Herbal teas, including chamomile, peppermint, and ginger, have an alkalizing effect on the body. They are soothing and hydrating, promoting relaxation and aiding digestion.

7. Alkaline Water:

- Alkaline water, with its increased pH level, can help neutralize excess acidity in the body. It is believed to have antioxidant properties and may support hydration and detoxification.

Nutritional Benefits of Alkaline Foods

Incorporating alkaline foods into your diet can provide numerous nutritional benefits. Here are some key advantages:

1. Improved Digestion:
   - Alkaline foods are typically rich in dietary fiber, which promotes regular bowel movements and supports a healthy digestive system. They can help alleviate issues like constipation and maintain a healthy gut.

2. Bone Health:
   - Many alkaline foods, such as leafy greens and root vegetables, are excellent sources of calcium, magnesium, and other minerals necessary for maintaining strong bones and reducing the risk of osteoporosis.

3. Reduced Inflammation:
   - An alkaline diet is often associated with reduced inflammation in the body. Chronic inflammation has been linked to various health conditions, including

heart disease, diabetes, and certain cancers. Alkaline foods, particularly fruits and vegetables, are rich in antioxidants and phytonutrients that help combat inflammation.

4. Increased Energy Levels:
   - Alkaline foods are nutrient-dense and provide a sustainable source of energy. They contain essential vitamins, minerals, and antioxidants that support overall vitality and combat fatigue.

5. pH Balance:
    - Consuming alkaline foods can help balance the body's pH levels. Excess acidity in the body can disrupt various bodily functions and contribute to health issues. Alkaline foods help neutralize acid, promoting a more balanced pH environment

Tips for Incorporating More Alkaline Foods into Your Diet

Incorporating alkaline foods into your diet is a great way to support your overall health and well-being. Here are some tips to help you incorporate more alkaline foods into your daily meals:

1. Start with Awareness:
    - Begin by familiarizing yourself with the list of alkaline foods mentioned earlier. Take note of the ones you enjoy and those you'd like to try. This awareness will guide you when planning your meals.

2. Increase Vegetable Intake:
    - Vegetables are the foundation of an alkaline diet. Aim to include a variety of leafy greens and cruciferous vegetables in your meals. Consider having a large salad with mixed greens as a side dish or adding steamed broccoli or cauliflower to your main course.

3. Choose Alkaline Fruits:
   - Incorporate alkaline fruits like lemons, limes, and grapefruits into your daily routine. Squeeze fresh lemon or lime juice over salads, vegetables, or in a glass of water. Enjoy a grapefruit as a snack or in a refreshing fruit salad.

4. Make Alkaline Snacks:
   - Nuts and seeds make excellent alkaline snacks. Keep a stash of almonds, pumpkin seeds, or chia seeds handy for a quick and nutritious snack option. You can also create homemade energy balls or bars using alkaline ingredients.

5. Experiment with Herbal Teas:
   - Replace caffeinated beverages with alkaline herbal teas. Explore different flavors such as chamomile, peppermint, or ginger. These teas not only have an alkalizing effect but also offer various health benefits.

6. Swap Processed Foods for Whole Foods:
   - Processed foods are typically acidic and can disrupt the body's pH balance. Opt for whole foods instead, such as whole grains, legumes, and fresh fruits and vegetables. These provide more alkalizing nutrients and are better for your health.

7. Plan Balanced Meals:
   - Create balanced meals that include alkaline foods along with other healthy components. Include a serving of alkaline

vegetables, a source of lean protein, and whole grains or legumes. This balance ensures you receive a wide range of nutrients.

8. Gradual Transition:
   - If you're new to incorporating alkaline foods, start gradually. Gradual changes are easier to sustain in the long run. Begin by adding one alkaline food at a time and gradually increase the variety and portion sizes.

9. Experiment with Recipes:
   - Explore recipes that focus on alkaline ingredients. Look for recipe ideas online or in cookbooks that feature alkaline foods as the main components. This can make your journey towards an alkaline diet more enjoyable and flavorful.

10. Stay Hydrated with Alkaline Water:
   - Hydration is essential for maintaining overall health. Consider drinking alkaline water to support your alkaline diet. You can purchase alkaline water or even make your own using water ionizers or alkaline drops.

Remember, while alkaline foods offer numerous health benefits, it's important to maintain a balanced and varied diet. Consult with a healthcare professional or a registered dietitian for personalized advice and guidance, especially if you have any specific health concerns or medical conditions.

Incorporating more alkaline foods into your diet can contribute to a healthier lifestyle and promote overall well-being. Enjoy the process of exploring new flavors and experimenting with alkaline ingredients in your meals. Your body will thank you for nourishing it with these nutrient-rich foods.

CHAPTER THREE

Acidic Foods to Avoid

List and Description of Acidic Foods

Acidic foods are those that have a low pH level, typically below 7.0 on the pH scale. These foods contain acids that can affect the acidity levels in our body. While some acidic foods can provide health benefits, consuming them in excess can have negative effects on our overall well-being. It's important to have a balanced diet and understand which acidic foods to include and limit in our daily meals. Here is a list and description of some common acidic foods:

1. Citrus Fruits: Citrus fruits like oranges, lemons, limes, and grapefruits are high in citric acid. They are acidic in nature but provide essential nutrients like vitamin C and fiber.

2. Tomatoes: Tomatoes are another acidic food due to their high malic and citric acid content. They are commonly used in salads, sauces, and various dishes. Tomatoes are also a good source of vitamins A and C.

3. Pineapple: Pineapple contains bromelain, an enzyme that aids in digestion. It is also rich in citric acid, making it an acidic fruit. Despite its acidity, pineapple offers several health benefits and is a good source of vitamins and minerals.

4. Vinegar: Various types of vinegar, such as apple cider vinegar, white vinegar, and balsamic vinegar, are acidic in nature. They add flavor to foods and are often used in dressings, marinades, and sauces.

5. Berries: Berries like strawberries, blueberries, raspberries, and blackberries are mildly acidic. They are also packed with antioxidants, vitamins, and fiber, making them a nutritious addition to your diet.

6. Fermented Foods: Fermented foods like yogurt, pickles, sauerkraut, and kimchi have a tangy taste due to the presence of lactic acid. These foods undergo fermentation, which promotes the growth of beneficial bacteria in our gut.

7. Coffee: While coffee itself is not acidic, it can stimulate the production of stomach acid, leading to acid reflux or heartburn. It's recommended to consume coffee in moderation, especially for individuals with digestive issues.

8. Carbonated Drinks: Soft drinks, energy drinks, and carbonated water are highly acidic due to the carbonation process. They contain phosphoric acid and citric acid, which can erode tooth enamel and contribute to dental problems.

9. Processed Meats: Processed meats like sausages,

bacon, and deli meats are often high in nitrates and phosphates, making them acidic. These meats have been linked to various health concerns and are best consumed in moderation.

10. Alcohol: Alcoholic beverages like wine, beer, and spirits can be acidic and may irritate the stomach lining. Excessive alcohol consumption can lead to gastritis, acid reflux, and other digestive issues.

It's worth noting that the acidity of a food doesn't necessarily determine its impact on our body's pH levels. Our body has its own mechanisms to maintain a balanced pH, and the overall dietary pattern plays a more significant role in this regard.

Negative Effects of Consuming Acidic Foods

While some acidic foods can be part of a healthy diet, excessive consumption or reliance on highly acidic foods can have negative effects on our health. Here are some potential negative effects of consuming acidic foods:

1. Acid Reflux: Acidic foods can trigger or worsen symptoms of acid reflux, a condition characterized by heartburn, regurgitation, and discomfort in the chest. Acid reflux occurs when stomach acid flows back into the esophagus, causing irritation and inflammation. Consuming

excessive amounts of acidic foods can increase the risk of acid reflux episodes.

2. Dental Issues: High consumption of acidic foods and beverages can erode tooth enamel over time. The acids in these foods weaken the protective layer of the teeth, making them more susceptible to decay and cavities. It's essential to practice good oral hygiene and limit the intake of acidic foods to protect dental health.

3. Digestive Discomfort: Some individuals may experience digestive discomfort, such as bloating, gas, and stomach pain, after consuming acidic foods. This is especially true for those with sensitive digestive systems or pre-existing digestive conditions like gastritis or irritable bowel syndrome (IBS).

4. Bone Health Concerns: The excessive intake of acidic foods may have an impact on bone health. When our body digests acidic foods, it uses alkaline minerals, such as calcium, to neutralize the acidity. Over time, this can lead to a depletion of calcium stores, potentially affecting bone density and increasing the risk of osteoporosis.

5. Imbalance in Gut Microbiota: The gut microbiota plays a crucial role in our overall health, including digestion, immune function, and mental well-being. Excessive consumption of acidic foods can disrupt the balance of beneficial bacteria in the gut, leading to gastrointestinal issues and compromising immune function.

6. Inflammation: Acidic foods can contribute to

an inflammatory response in the body. Chronic inflammation has been associated with various health conditions, including cardiovascular disease, diabetes, and certain types of cancer. While acidic foods alone may not be the sole cause of inflammation, a diet high in acidic foods and low in anti-inflammatory foods can contribute to an imbalance.

Strategies for Reducing or Eliminating Acidic Foods from Your Diet

If you're concerned about the negative effects of consuming acidic foods or wish to reduce your intake for other reasons, here are some strategies to help you:

1. Awareness and Education: Start by educating yourself about the pH levels and acidity of different foods. Familiarize yourself with the list of acidic foods and their potential impact on your health. This knowledge will help you make informed choices and develop a well-balanced diet.

2. Balance and Moderation: Instead of completely eliminating acidic foods, strive for a balanced approach. Incorporate a variety of foods from different pH levels into your meals. Combine acidic foods with alkaline-rich foods, such as leafy greens, to create a more neutral balance. Moderation is key, as consuming acidic foods in moderate amounts is generally well-tolerated by most individuals.

3. Meal Planning and Preparation: Plan your meals in advance to ensure a well-rounded and diverse diet. Incorporate a variety of fruits, vegetables, whole grains, and lean proteins. When cooking, opt for methods that require less added acidity, such as grilling, steaming, or baking, instead of using acidic sauces or dressings.

4. Substitutions and Alternatives: Explore substitutions for highly acidic ingredients. For example, use herbs, spices, and vinegar-free dressings to add flavor to your dishes. Replace carbonated drinks with infused water, herbal teas, or natural fruit juices. Experiment with non-acidic fruits like bananas, melons, and avocados as alternatives to highly acidic fruits.

5. Hydration and Alkaline Foods: Stay adequately hydrated by consuming plenty of water throughout the day. Drinking water helps maintain proper pH balance in the body. Additionally, include alkaline-rich foods in your diet, such as leafy greens, cucumbers, celery, and almonds. These foods have a higher alkaline content, which can help counterbalance the acidity in your body.

6. Mindful Eating: Practice mindful eating by paying attention to your body's cues and listening to its signals of hunger and fullness. This can help you make conscious choices about the foods you consume. Slow down during meals, chew your food thoroughly, and savor the flavors. By doing so, you may naturally eat less and be more aware of the impact of acidic foods on your body.

7. Seek Professional Advice: If you have specific health concerns or dietary restrictions, it's advisable to consult a healthcare professional or registered dietitian. They can provide personalized guidance and recommendations tailored to your individual needs.

8. Keep a Food Diary: Keeping a food diary can help you track your consumption of acidic foods and identify any patterns or triggers. This can be useful if you suspect that certain acidic foods are causing negative effects on your health. By documenting your meals and symptoms, you can work with a healthcare professional to make informed decisions about your diet.

9. Gradual Changes: If you're considering eliminating or reducing acidic foods from your diet, it's often more sustainable to make gradual changes rather than implementing drastic restrictions. Start by gradually reducing the portion sizes or frequency of acidic foods and gradually replacing them with healthier alternatives. This approach allows your body and taste buds to adjust more easily.

10. Focus on Overall Diet Quality: While it's important to be mindful of acidic foods, it's equally crucial to focus on the overall quality of your diet. Aim for a well-balanced, varied diet that includes plenty of fruits, vegetables, whole grains, lean proteins, and healthy fats. Prioritize nutrient-dense foods that support your overall health and well-being.

CHAPTER FOUR

Tips for Maintaining an Alkaline Diet on a Daily Basis

Maintaining an alkaline diet can have numerous health benefits, including improved digestion, increased energy levels, and reduced inflammation. The concept behind an alkaline diet is to consume foods that help balance the body's pH levels and promote overall well-being. Here are some tips to help you maintain an alkaline diet on a daily basis.

1. Focus on Plant-Based Foods

One of the fundamental principles of an alkaline diet is to emphasize plant-based foods. Include a variety of fruits and vegetables in your daily meals, as they are generally alkaline-forming in the body. Leafy greens, such as kale, spinach, and Swiss chard, are excellent choices.

Other alkaline-rich options include broccoli, cucumbers, avocados, and bell peppers. Aim to fill at least half of your plate with these alkaline vegetables.

2. Choose Alkaline Protein Sources

While plant-based proteins are generally more alkaline, you can still incorporate some animal proteins into an alkaline diet. Opt for lean sources like fish, chicken, and turkey. These proteins are less acidic compared to red meat and can be included in moderation. Additionally, plant-based protein sources such as lentils, quinoa, and tofu are excellent choices for an alkaline diet.

3. Reduce Acidic Foods

To maintain an alkaline diet, it is important to reduce the consumption of acidic foods. Acidic foods can disrupt the body's pH balance and lead to increased acidity. Some common acidic foods include processed meats, refined grains, sugary snacks, and carbonated beverages. Limiting the intake of these foods can help maintain a more alkaline state in your body.

4. Stay Hydrated

Proper hydration is crucial for maintaining an alkaline diet. Drinking enough water helps flush out toxins and supports optimal body functions. Aim to drink at least eight glasses of water per day. Consider adding a squeeze of lemon to your water as it can have an alkalizing effect on the body. Additionally, herbal teas, such as chamomile or green tea, can also contribute to your daily fluid intake.

5. Practice Mindful Eating

Practicing mindful eating can help you maintain an alkaline diet more effectively. Slow down and pay attention to your meals. Chew your food thoroughly and savor each bite. This allows for better digestion and absorption of nutrients. Avoid eating in front of screens or while multitasking, as it can lead to mindless eating and overconsumption of acidic foods.

6. Plan and Prepare Your Meals

Planning and preparing your meals in advance can

significantly contribute to maintaining an alkaline diet. Set aside time each week to plan your meals and create a shopping list. Include alkaline foods and recipes that align with your dietary goals. Preparing your meals at home gives you better control over the ingredients and ensures you have alkaline options readily available.

7. Incorporate Alkaline Snacks

Snacking can be a challenge when following an alkaline diet, as many convenient snack options are acidic. However, there are several alkaline snacks that you can enjoy. Raw nuts and seeds, such as almonds, walnuts, and chia seeds, are great choices. Fresh fruits like apples, berries, and grapes are also alkaline-rich snacks. Prepare homemade vegetable sticks with hummus or guacamole for a satisfying and alkaline snack option.

8. Be Mindful of Acid-Alkaline Balance

While following an alkaline diet, it is important to be mindful of the acid-alkaline balance in your meals. The goal is to consume a higher proportion of alkaline-forming foods while minimizing acidic foods. It's not necessary to completely eliminate acidic foods, as some are still beneficial in moderation. Strive for balance and aim for a diet that consists of approximately 70-80% alkaline-forming foods and 20-30% acidic foods.

9. Experiment with Alkaline Recipes

Maintaining an alkaline diet doesn't mean sacrificing flavor and variety. There are plenty of delicious alkaline recipes available that can help you stay on track. Explore different recipes that incorporate alkaline ingredients like quinoa, lentils, leafy greens, and colorful vegetables. Experiment with herbs and spices to enhance the taste of your dishes without relying on excessive salt or acidic sauces. Look for online resources or alkaline cookbooks for inspiration.

10. Educate Yourself

To successfully maintain an alkaline diet, it's important to educate yourself about the principles and benefits of this lifestyle. Learn about the pH levels of different foods, the impact of acidity on the body, and the science behind alkaline diets. Understanding the reasoning behind the diet can help you stay motivated and make informed choices about the foods you consume. Consult reputable sources, books, or seek guidance from a registered dietitian specializing in alkaline diets.

Importance of Regular Hydration and Alkaline Water

Hydration plays a vital role in overall health, and incorporating alkaline water into your daily routine can provide additional benefits. Here's why regular hydration and alkaline water are important:

1. Maintaining Optimal Hydration

Proper hydration is essential for various bodily functions, including digestion, circulation, temperature regulation, and nutrient absorption. Water is necessary for the body to function optimally, and being adequately hydrated can help improve energy levels, support brain function, and promote healthy skin.

2. Alkaline Water and pH Balance

Alkaline water has a higher pH level than regular tap water, typically ranging from 8 to 9.5. Consuming alkaline water can help counterbalance the acidity that may accumulate in the body due to dietary and lifestyle factors. It is believed that alkaline water can help restore pH balance, promote detoxification, and reduce the risk of chronic diseases associated with high acidity levels.

3. Enhanced Hydration and Electrolyte Balance

Alkaline water often contains essential minerals such as calcium, potassium, and magnesium, which are important for maintaining electrolyte balance in the body. These minerals can contribute to better hydration by improving water absorption at the cellular level. Additionally, alkaline water is often less acidic than regular water, which can make it easier to drink and potentially enhance overall hydration.

Incorporating Alkaline Principles into Other Aspects of Life

Maintaining an alkaline lifestyle extends beyond just

dietary choices. Here are some tips for incorporating alkaline principles into other aspects of life, including exercise and stress management:

1. Exercise and Physical Activity

Regular exercise is crucial for overall health and can complement an alkaline diet. Engage in activities that you enjoy, such as walking, jogging, swimming, or yoga. Exercise helps improve circulation, supports detoxification, and reduces stress levels, all of which can contribute to a more alkaline state in the body. Aim for at least 30 minutes of moderate-intensity exercise most days of the week.

2. Stress Management and Mindfulness

Stress can contribute to acidity in the body, so incorporating stress management techniques and mindfulness practices can help maintain an alkaline state. Explore relaxation techniques such as deep breathing exercises, meditation, or yoga to reduce stress levels. Engaging in activities that bring you joy and practicing self-care can also have a positive impact on your overall well-being and support alkaline principles.

3. Prioritize Quality Sleep

Adequate sleep is crucial for maintaining a healthy alkaline balance. During sleep, the body repairs and rejuvenates itself. Aim for 7-9 hours of quality sleep each night to support overall health and well-being. Establish a relaxing bedtime routine, create a comfortable sleep environment, and limit exposure to electronic devices before bed to promote restful sleep.

4. Mindful Exposure to Nature

Connecting with nature and spending time outdoors can have alkaline-promoting effects on the body and mind. Take regular walks in nature, engage in gardening, or simply spend time in green spaces. Fresh air, sunlight, and being in natural surroundings can reduce stress levels and improve mood, contributing to an alkaline lifestyle.

5. Practice Gratitude and Positive Thinking

Cultivating a positive mindset and practicing gratitude can help reduce stress and promote alkaline principles. Take time each day to reflect on things you are grateful for and focus on positive aspects of your life. Surround yourself with supportive and positive individuals who uplift your spirits and share in your alkaline journey.

6. Limit Exposure to Toxins

Toxins from various sources, including environmental pollutants and chemical-laden personal care products, can contribute to acidity in the body. Minimize exposure to toxins by opting for natural and organic products, using non-toxic cleaning supplies, and being mindful of the air quality in your living spaces. This conscious effort to reduce toxin exposure supports an alkaline lifestyle and overall well-being.

7. Seek Balance in Relationships

Maintaining healthy relationships and nurturing a positive social network is an essential aspect of an alkaline lifestyle. Surround yourself with supportive individuals who encourage your alkaline journey and share similar health goals. Seek balance in your relationships, setting boundaries when necessary, and fostering connections that bring joy, positivity, and support into your life.

Incorporating alkaline principles into various aspects of life beyond just diet can help promote overall well-being and support a more alkaline state in the body. By prioritizing hydration, mindful eating, stress management, exercise, and positive lifestyle choices, you can create a holistic alkaline lifestyle that contributes to your long-term health and vitality.

CHAPTEER FIVE

Recipes and Meal Plans

Sample alkaline recipes for breakfast

Alkaline Green Smoothie Bowl

Description: This Alkaline Green Smoothie Bowl is a refreshing and nutritious breakfast option. Packed with vibrant green fruits and vegetables, it provides a burst of energy to start your day on a healthy note.

Ingredients:

- 1 ripe banana
- 1 cup spinach leaves
- 1/2 avocado
- 1/2 cucumber
- 1/2 cup almond milk
- 1 tablespoon chia seeds
- 1 tablespoon hemp seeds
- 1 tablespoon almond butter
- 1 teaspoon spirulina powder (optional)

- Fresh berries and sliced fruits for topping

Instructions:

1. In a blender, combine the ripe banana, spinach leaves, avocado, cucumber, almond milk, chia seeds, hemp seeds, almond butter, and spirulina powder (if using). Blend until smooth and creamy.

2. Pour the smoothie mixture into a bowl.

3. Top with fresh berries and sliced fruits of your choice.

4. Enjoy immediately.

Nutritional Information: This smoothie bowl is rich in fiber, healthy fats, vitamins, and minerals. It provides a good amount of potassium, vitamin C, vitamin K, and antioxidants. The exact nutritional content may vary depending on the specific brands and quantities of ingredients used.

Quinoa Breakfast Porridge

Description: This Quinoa Breakfast Porridge is a hearty and nutritious meal that will keep you satisfied throughout the morning. Quinoa, a complete protein, is combined with warming spices and topped with nuts and fruits for a delicious start to your day.

Ingredients:

- 1/2 cup quinoa
- 1 cup almond milk
- 1/2 teaspoon cinnamon
- 1/4 teaspoon nutmeg
- 1/4 teaspoon vanilla extract
- 1 tablespoon maple syrup (optional)
- Assorted nuts, seeds, and fruits for topping

Instructions:

1. Rinse the quinoa under cold water to remove any bitterness.

2. In a saucepan, combine the rinsed quinoa, almond milk, cinnamon, nutmeg, and vanilla extract. Bring to a boil over medium heat.

3. Reduce the heat to low and simmer for about 15-20 minutes, or until the quinoa is cooked and the porridge has thickened to your desired consistency. Stir occasionally to prevent sticking.

4. Remove from heat and stir in the maple syrup, if using.

5. Serve the quinoa porridge in bowls and top with your choice of assorted nuts, seeds, and fruits.

6. Enjoy while warm.

Nutritional Information: This quinoa breakfast porridge is a good source of plant-based protein, dietary fiber, and essential minerals such as magnesium and phosphorus. It provides sustained energy and is a great option for those following a gluten-free or vegetarian diet.

Alkaline Avocado Toast

Description: Alkaline Avocado Toast is a simple and delicious breakfast or snack option that is both satisfying and nutritious. Creamy avocado spread on top of toasted bread creates a perfect combination of flavors and textures.

Ingredients:

- 2 slices whole grain bread
- 1 ripe avocado
- 1 tablespoon lemon juice
- Pinch of sea salt
- Pinch of black pepper
- Optional toppings: sliced tomatoes, sprouts, red pepper flakes

Instructions:

1. Toast the slices of whole grain bread until golden

and crispy.

2. While the bread is toasting, cut the ripe avocado in half and remove the pit. Scoop the flesh into a bowl.

3. Add the lemon juice, sea salt, and black pepper to the bowl with the avocado. Mash and mix well until you achieve a creamy consistency. 4

4. Once the bread is toasted, spread the mashed avocado mixture evenly on each slice.

4. If desired, add additional toppings such as sliced tomatoes, sprouts, or a sprinkle of red pepper flakes for extra flavor and texture.

5. Serve the avocado toast immediately and enjoy it as a nutritious breakfast or snack.

Nutritional Information: Alkaline Avocado Toast provides a good amount of healthy fats, dietary fiber, and vitamins. Avocado is a rich source of monounsaturated fats, which are beneficial for heart health. The whole grain bread adds complex carbohydrates and fiber to help keep you satisfied and energized.

Alkaline Chia Pudding

Description: Alkaline Chia Pudding is a creamy and indulgent dessert-like breakfast option that is packed with nutrition. Chia seeds, known for their high omega-3 fatty acid content, are soaked in almond milk to create a thick and pudding-like consistency.

Ingredients:

- 2 tablespoons chia seeds
- 1 cup almond milk
- 1/2 teaspoon vanilla extract
- 1 tablespoon maple syrup (optional)
- Fresh fruits, nuts, or seeds for topping

Instructions:

1. In a bowl, combine the chia seeds, almond milk, vanilla extract, and maple syrup (if desired). Stir well to ensure the chia seeds are evenly distributed.

2. Let the mixture sit for about 5 minutes, then stir again to prevent clumping.

3. Cover the bowl and refrigerate for at least 2 hours or overnight to allow the chia seeds to absorb the liquid and thicken into a pudding-like consistency.

4. Before serving, give the chia pudding a good stir to break up any clumps.

5. Divide the pudding into individual serving dishes and top with fresh fruits, nuts, or seeds of your choice.

6. Enjoy the Alkaline Chia Pudding as a nourishing and satisfying breakfast or snack.

Nutritional Information: Alkaline Chia Pudding is rich in omega-3 fatty acids, dietary fiber, and calcium. Chia seeds are also a good source of antioxidants and protein. This pudding is low in added sugars and can be customized with a variety of toppings to suit your taste preferences.

Alkaline Vegetable Omelette

Description: Alkaline Vegetable Omelette is a protein-packed breakfast option that combines the goodness of eggs with a variety of colorful vegetables. It is a nutritious and delicious way to start your day.

Ingredients:

- 2 large eggs
- 1/4 cup chopped bell peppers (any color)
- 1/4 cup chopped spinach
- 1/4 cup sliced mushrooms
- 1/4 cup diced tomatoes
- 1/4 cup diced onions
- 1 tablespoon olive oil
- Pinch of sea salt

- Pinch of black pepper

Instructions:

- In a bowl, beat the eggs until well mixed. Season with a pinch of sea salt and black pepper.
- Heat the olive oil in a non-stick skillet over medium heat.
- Add the onions and bell peppers to the skillet and sauté for 2-3 minutes until slightly softened.
- Add the mushrooms and spinach to the skillet and continue to sauté for another 2-3 minutes until the vegetables are tender.
- Pour the beaten eggs over the sautéed vegetables in the skillet. Allow the eggs to cook undisturbed for a few minutes until the edges start to set.
- Gently lift the edges of the omelette with a spatula and tilt the skillet to let the uncooked eggs flow to the edges.

- Cook the omelette for a few more minutes until the bottom is set and the top is slightly runny.
- Carefully fold one side of the omelette over the other to create a half-moon shape.
- Cook for another minute to ensure the eggs are fully cooked.
- Slide the omelette onto a plate and garnish with diced tomatoes.
- Serve the Alkaline Vegetable Omelette hot and enjoy it as a nutritious breakfast or brunch option.

Nutritional Information: Alkaline Vegetable Omelette is

a great source of high-quality protein, vitamins, and minerals. Eggs provide essential amino acids and nutrients such as vitamin B12, vitamin D, and choline. The colorful assortment of vegetables adds fiber, antioxidants, and a variety of vitamins and minerals.

Almond Butter and Banana Wrap

Description: Almond Butter and Banana Wrap is a quick and satisfying breakfast or snack option that combines the creaminess of almond butter with the natural sweetness of bananas. It's a delightful combination wrapped in a tortilla for a portable and nutritious meal.

Ingredients:

- 1 whole wheat tortilla
- 2 tablespoons almond butter
- 1 ripe banana, sliced
- Optional toppings: honey, chia seeds, shredded coconut

Instructions:

1. Lay the whole wheat tortilla on a flat surface.
2. Spread the almond butter evenly over the tortilla.

3. Place the sliced banana in a row down the center of the tortilla.

4. If desired, drizzle a small amount of honey over the bananas and sprinkle with chia seeds or shredded coconut.

5. Fold in the sides of the tortilla and roll it up tightly, like a burrito.

6. Slice the wrap in half diagonally, if desired, for easier handling.

7. Enjoy the Almond Butter and Banana Wrap as a quick and nutritious breakfast on the go or as a satisfying snack.

Nutritional Information: Almond Butter and Banana Wrap provides a balance of carbohydrates, healthy fats, and natural sugars. Almond butter is a good source of protein, healthy fats, and vitamin E, while bananas offer potassium, vitamin C, and dietary fiber. The whole wheat tortilla adds complex carbohydrates and additional fiber.

Blueberry Almond Pancakes

Description: Blueberry Almond Pancakes are fluffy, flavorful, and bursting with juicy blueberries. These pancakes are made with almond flour, providing a gluten-free and nutrient-rich alternative to traditional pancakes.

Ingredients:

- 1 cup almond flour
- 2 tablespoons coconut flour
- 1 teaspoon baking powder
- 1/4 teaspoon salt
- 2 large eggs
- 1/2 cup almond milk
- 1 tablespoon maple syrup (optional)
- 1/2 teaspoon vanilla extract
- 1/2 cup fresh blueberries
- Coconut oil for greasing the pan

Instructions:

1. In a large mixing bowl, whisk together the almond flour, coconut flour, baking powder, and salt.

2. In a separate bowl, beat the eggs. Add almond milk, maple syrup (if using), and vanilla extract. Mix well.

3. Pour the wet ingredients into the dry ingredients and stir until just combined. Be careful not to overmix.

4. Gently fold in the fresh blueberries.

5. Heat a non-stick skillet or griddle over medium heat and lightly grease with coconut oil.

6. Pour 1/4 cup of the pancake batter onto the skillet for each pancake.

7. Cook for 2-3 minutes, or until bubbles start to form on the surface. Flip the pancakes and cook for an additional 2-3 minutes, or until golden brown and cooked through.

8. Repeat with the remaining batter, adding more coconut oil to the skillet as needed.

9. Serve the Blueberry Almond Pancakes warm, topped with additional fresh blueberries and a drizzle of maple syrup if desired.

Nutritional Information: Blueberry Almond Pancakes are a nutritious and gluten-free option for a delightful breakfast. Almond flour provides healthy fats, protein, and vitamin E, while blueberries offer antioxidants and vitamins. These pancakes are lower in carbohydrates compared to traditional pancakes, making them suitable for those following a low-carb or gluten-free diet.

Lunch

Alkaline Chickpea Salad

Description: Alkaline Chickpea Salad is a refreshing and nutritious dish that combines the goodness of chickpeas with a variety of colorful vegetables. This salad is packed with protein, fiber, and essential nutrients, making it a perfect choice for a healthy and satisfying meal.

Ingredients:

- 1 can chickpeas, drained and rinsed
- 1 cup cherry tomatoes, halved
- 1 cucumber, diced
- 1 red bell pepper, diced
- 1/4 red onion, thinly sliced
- 1/4 cup fresh parsley, chopped
- 2 tablespoons olive oil
- 1 tablespoon lemon juice
- Salt and pepper to taste

Instructions:

1. In a large bowl, combine the chickpeas, cherry tomatoes, cucumber, red bell pepper, red onion, and fresh parsley.

2. In a small bowl, whisk together the olive oil, lemon juice, salt, and pepper.

3. Pour the dressing over the salad and toss gently to coat all the ingredients.

4. Refrigerate for at least 30 minutes to allow the flavors to meld together.

5. Serve chilled and enjoy!

Nutritional Information:

- Serving Size: 1 cup
- Calories: 180
- Total Fat: 8g
- Saturated Fat: 1g
- Sodium: 180mg
- Carbohydrates: 22g
- Fiber: 6g
- Protein: 6g

Quinoa and Roasted Vegetable Bowl

Description: Quinoa and Roasted Vegetable Bowl is a hearty and nutritious meal that combines fluffy quinoa with a medley of roasted vegetables. This bowl is packed with vitamins, minerals, and fiber, providing a satisfying and wholesome dining experience.

Ingredients:

- 1 cup quinoa
- 2 cups vegetable broth
- 1 small sweet potato, diced
- 1 zucchini, sliced
- 1 red bell pepper, sliced
- 1 cup broccoli florets
- 2 tablespoons olive oil
- 1 teaspoon dried thyme

- 1/2 teaspoon garlic powder
- Salt and pepper to taste

Instructions:

1. Preheat the oven to 425°F (220°C).

2. Rinse the quinoa under cold water and drain.

3. In a medium saucepan, bring the vegetable broth to a boil. Add the quinoa, reduce the heat to low, cover, and simmer for 15-20 minutes or until the liquid is absorbed and the quinoa is tender. Fluff with a fork and set aside.

4. In a large baking sheet, toss the sweet potato, zucchini, red bell pepper, and broccoli florets with olive oil, dried thyme, garlic powder, salt, and pepper.

5. Roast the vegetables in the preheated oven for 20-25 minutes or until they are tender and slightly caramelized.

6. In a serving bowl, layer the cooked quinoa and roasted vegetables.

7. Serve warm and enjoy!

Nutritional Information:

- Serving Size: 1 bowl
- Calories: 320
- Total Fat: 10g
- Saturated Fat: 1.5g
- Sodium: 480mg

- Carbohydrates: 50g
- Fiber: 8g
- Protein: 10g

Alkaline Lentil Soup

Description: Alkaline Lentil Soup is a comforting and nourishing dish that combines the goodness of lentils with aromatic herbs and spices. This soup is rich in protein, fiber, and essential nutrients, making it a satisfying and healthy option for a meal.

Ingredients:

- 1 cup dried lentils
- 4 cups vegetable broth
- 1 onion, chopped
- 2 carrots, diced
- 2 celery stalks, diced
- 3 garlic cloves, minced
- 1 teaspoon ground cumin
- 1 teaspoon ground turmeric
- 1/2 teaspoon paprika
- Salt and pepper to taste
- Fresh parsley for garnish

Instructions:

1. Rinse the lentils under cold water and drain.

2. In a large pot, heat some olive oil over medium heat. Add the chopped onion, carrots, and celery, and sauté until they become tender, about 5 minutes.

3. Add the minced garlic, cumin, turmeric, paprika, salt, and pepper. Stir well to coat the vegetables in the spices.

4. Add the lentils to the pot and pour in the vegetable broth. Bring to a boil, then reduce the heat to low and simmer for about 30-40 minutes or until the lentils are cooked and tender.

5. Taste the soup and adjust the seasoning if needed.

6. Ladle the soup into bowls, garnish with fresh parsley, and serve hot.

Nutritional Information:

- Serving Size: 1 cup
- Calories: 180
- Total Fat: 1g
- Saturated Fat: 0g
- Sodium: 480mg
- Carbohydrates: 32g
- Fiber: 15g
- Protein: 12g

Spinach and Avocado Salad

Description: Spinach and Avocado Salad is a light and refreshing dish that combines the vibrant flavors of fresh spinach, creamy avocado, and tangy dressing. This salad is packed with vitamins, minerals, and healthy fats, making it a nutritious and delicious choice.

Ingredients:

- 4 cups fresh spinach leaves
- 1 ripe avocado, sliced
- 1 cup cherry tomatoes, halved
- 1/4 red onion, thinly sliced
- 2 tablespoons lemon juice
- 2 tablespoons extra virgin olive oil
- 1 tablespoon honey
- Salt and pepper to taste

Instructions:

1. In a large bowl, combine the fresh spinach leaves, sliced avocado, cherry tomatoes, and thinly sliced red onion.

2. In a small bowl, whisk together the lemon juice, extra virgin olive oil, honey, salt, and pepper to make the dressing.

3. Drizzle the dressing over the salad and toss gently to coat all the ingredients.

4. Serve immediately and enjoy the vibrant flavors!

Nutritional Information:

- Serving Size: 1 cup
- Calories: 160
- Total Fat: 12g
- Saturated Fat: 2g
- Sodium: 70mg
- Carbohydrates: 12g
- Fiber: 6g
- Protein: 4g

Alkaline Veggie Wrap

Description: Alkaline Veggie Wrap is a flavorful and nutritious meal that features a variety of fresh vegetables wrapped in a whole wheat tortilla. This wrap is packed with fiber, vitamins, and minerals, making it a satisfying and healthy choice for a quick lunch or dinner.

Ingredients:

- 1 whole wheat tortilla
- 1/2 cup hummus
- 1/4 cup shredded carrots
- 1/4 cup sliced cucumbers
- 1/4 cup sliced bell peppers
- 1/4 cup baby spinach leaves

- 1/4 cup sprouts
- Salt and pepper to taste

Instructions:

1. Lay the whole wheat tortilla on a clean surface and spread the hummus evenly over the tortilla. 2. Layer the shredded carrots, sliced cucumbers, bell peppers, baby spinach leaves, and sprouts on top of the hummus.

3. Sprinkle with salt and pepper to taste.

4. Tightly roll up the tortilla, folding in the sides as you go.

5. Slice the wrap in half diagonally to make it easier to eat, if desired.

6. Serve immediately or wrap in foil for a convenient grab-and-go meal.

Nutritional Information:

- Serving Size: 1 wrap
- Calories: 280
- Total Fat: 10g
- Saturated Fat: 1g
- Sodium: 520mg
- Carbohydrates: 38g
- Fiber: 9g
- Protein: 10g

Almond Crusted Tofu with Stir-Fried Vegetables

Description: Almond Crusted Tofu with Stir-Fried Vegetables is a delicious and protein-packed dish that combines crispy almond-crusted tofu with a medley of colorful stir-fried vegetables. This meal is full of flavor and provides a balanced combination of plant-based protein, healthy fats, and a variety of nutrients.

Ingredients:

- 1 block of firm tofu, drained and pressed
- 1/2 cup almond meal
- 2 tablespoons cornstarch
- 1/2 teaspoon garlic powder
- 1/2 teaspoon paprika
- Salt and pepper to taste
- 2 tablespoons olive oil, divided
- 1 red bell pepper, thinly sliced
- 1 zucchini, thinly sliced
- 1 carrot, thinly sliced
- 1 cup broccoli florets
- 2 tablespoons soy sauce
- 1 tablespoon rice vinegar
- 1 teaspoon sesame oil
- Optional toppings: sesame seeds, green onions

Instructions:

1. Preheat the oven to 400°F (200°C).

2. Cut the tofu into rectangular slices, about 1/2 inch thick.

3. In a shallow dish, combine the almond meal, cornstarch, garlic powder, paprika, salt, and pepper.

4. Dip each tofu slice into the almond mixture, pressing gently to coat both sides.

5. Heat 1 tablespoon of olive oil in a large skillet over medium heat. Add the coated tofu slices and cook until golden brown and crispy on both sides, about 3-4 minutes per side. Transfer the tofu to a baking sheet lined with parchment paper.

6. Place the tofu in the preheated oven and bake for 10-12 minutes to further crisp up.

7. In the same skillet, heat the remaining tablespoon of olive oil. Add the sliced bell pepper, zucchini, carrot, and broccoli florets. Stir-fry for 5-6 minutes until the vegetables are tender-crisp.

8. In a small bowl, whisk together the soy sauce, rice vinegar, and sesame oil. Pour the sauce over the stir-fried vegetables and toss to coat.

9. Serve the almond-crusted tofu alongside the stir-fried vegetables. Garnish with sesame seeds and green onions if desired.

Nutritional Information:

- Serving Size: 1/2 tofu block with stir-fried vegetables
- Calories: 380

- Total Fat: 22g
- Saturated Fat: 2.5g
- Sodium: 560mg
- Carbohydrates: 27g
- Fiber: 7g
- Protein: 24g

Dinner

Alkaline Zucchini Noodles with Pesto

Description: This refreshing and light dish combines the freshness of zucchini noodles with a flavorful pesto sauce. It's a perfect choice for a healthy and vibrant meal.

Ingredients:

- 3 medium zucchinis
- 1 cup fresh basil leaves
- 1/4 cup pine nuts
- 2 cloves garlic
- 1/4 cup extra-virgin olive oil
- 1 tablespoon lemon juice
- Salt and pepper to taste
- Optional toppings: cherry tomatoes, sliced avocado

Instructions:

1. Using a spiralizer or a vegetable peeler, create zucchini noodles by cutting the zucchinis into thin, noodle-like strips.

2. In a food processor, combine the basil leaves, pine nuts, garlic, olive oil, lemon juice, salt, and pepper. Process until the mixture becomes a smooth pesto sauce.

3. In a large skillet, heat some olive oil over medium heat. Add the zucchini noodles and cook for about 2-3 minutes until they are slightly tender.

4. Pour the pesto sauce over the zucchini noodles and toss gently to coat them evenly.

5. Cook for an additional 2 minutes until the pesto is heated through.

6. Serve the zucchini noodles with optional toppings such as cherry tomatoes and sliced avocado.

7. Enjoy this flavorful and alkaline-packed meal!

Nutritional Information:

- Calories: 250
- Carbohydrates: 12g
- Protein: 5g
- Fat: 22g
- Fiber: 4g

Baked Lemon Herb Salmon with Roasted Asparagus

Description: This delicious and nutritious meal features tender baked salmon infused with zesty lemon and aromatic herbs, accompanied by roasted asparagus for a satisfying and healthy combination.

Ingredients:

- 4 salmon fillets
- 2 lemons, sliced
- 2 tablespoons chopped fresh dill
- 2 tablespoons chopped fresh parsley
- 2 cloves garlic, minced
- Salt and pepper to taste
- 1 bunch asparagus, trimmed
- 2 tablespoons olive oil

Instructions:

1. Preheat the oven to 400°F (200°C). Line a baking sheet with parchment paper.

2. Place the salmon fillets on the prepared baking sheet. Season them with salt, pepper, minced garlic, and chopped herbs (dill and parsley).

3. Arrange lemon slices on top of each salmon fillet.

4. In a separate bowl, toss the trimmed asparagus with olive oil, salt, and pepper.

5. Place the seasoned asparagus on the baking sheet alongside the salmon.

6. Bake in the preheated oven for about 12-15 minutes, or until the salmon is cooked through and flakes easily with a fork.

7. Serve the baked lemon herb salmon with roasted asparagus.

8. Enjoy this flavorful and nutritious meal!

Nutritional Information:

- Calories: 350
- Carbohydrates: 10g
- Protein: 30g
- Fat: 22g
- Fiber: 5g

Alkaline Cauliflower Rice Stir-Fry

Description: This stir-fry is a healthy and satisfying dish that replaces traditional rice with cauliflower rice. Packed with colorful vegetables and flavorful seasonings, it's a delicious way to enjoy a low-carb and alkaline meal.

Ingredients:

- 1 small head of cauliflower
- 1 tablespoon coconut oil
- 1 red bell pepper, thinly sliced
- 1 yellow bell pepper, thinly sliced

- 1 carrot, julienned
- 1 cup broccoli florets
- 1 cup snap peas, trimmed
- 2 cloves garlic, minced
- 2 tablespoons tamari sauce (or soy sauce for non-alkaline version)
- 1 tablespoon rice vinegar
- 1 tablespoon sesame oil
- Optional toppings: sesame seeds, chopped green onions

Instructions:

1. Cut the cauliflower into florets and pulse them in a food processor until they resemble rice-like grains. Set aside.

2. Heat the coconut oil in a large skillet or wok over medium heat.

3. Add the minced garlic and sauté for a minute until fragrant.

4. Add the sliced bell peppers, julienned carrot, broccoli florets, and snap peas to the skillet. Stir-fry for about 3-4 minutes until the vegetables are crisp-tender.

5. Push the vegetables to one side of the skillet and add the cauliflower rice to the other side.

6. Drizzle the tamari sauce, rice vinegar, and sesame oil over the cauliflower rice. Stir-fry everything together for an additional 2-3 minutes until the cauliflower rice is cooked but still slightly crisp.

7. Remove from heat and garnish with sesame seeds and chopped green onions, if desired.

8. Serve the alkaline cauliflower rice stir-fry as a satisfying and flavorful meal option.

Nutritional Information:

- Calories: 180
- Carbohydrates: 15g
- Protein: 7g
- Fat: 10g
- Fiber: 7g

Grilled Portobello Mushrooms with Quinoa Pilaf

Description: These hearty grilled portobello mushrooms are marinated in a flavorful sauce and served with a wholesome quinoa pilaf. This dish is packed with protein, fiber, and earthy flavors, making it a delicious and satisfying meal.

Ingredients:

- 4 large portobello mushrooms
- 2 tablespoons balsamic vinegar
- 2 tablespoons olive oil
- 2 cloves garlic, minced
- 1 tablespoon fresh thyme leaves

- Salt and pepper to taste
- 1 cup cooked quinoa
- 1/2 cup diced bell peppers (any color)
- 1/2 cup diced zucchini
- 1/4 cup chopped red onion
- 2 tablespoons lemon juice
- 2 tablespoons chopped fresh parsley

Instructions:

1. Preheat the grill to medium-high heat.

2. In a small bowl, whisk together balsamic vinegar, olive oil, minced garlic, thyme leaves, salt, and pepper to make the marinade.

3. Remove the stems from the portobello mushrooms and brush the marinade on both sides of the mushrooms.

4. Place the mushrooms on the grill, gill side down, and cook for about 5-6 minutes per side until they are tender and juicy.

5. While the mushrooms are grilling, prepare the quinoa pilaf. In a medium bowl, combine cooked quinoa, diced bell peppers, diced zucchini, chopped red onion, lemon juice, chopped parsley, salt, and pepper. Mix well.

6. Remove the grilled portobello mushrooms from the grill and let them rest for a few minutes.

7. Serve the mushrooms over a bed of quinoa pilaf.

8. Enjoy the deliciousness of grilled portobello mushrooms with nutritious quinoa pilaf.

Nutritional Information:

- Calories: 280
- Carbohydrates: 30g
- Protein: 10g
- Fat: 14g
- Fiber: 5g

Alkaline Black Bean and Sweet Potato Tacos

Description: These flavorful tacos feature a delicious combination of alkaline black beans and sweet potatoes, seasoned with aromatic spices and served in warm tortillas. They are a satisfying and wholesome meal option for any time of the day.

Ingredients:

- 1 tablespoon olive oil
- 1 small onion, diced
- 2 cloves garlic, minced
- 1 teaspoon ground cumin
- 1 teaspoon smoked paprika
- 1/2 teaspoon chili powder
- 2 cups cooked black beans
- 1 large sweet potato, peeled and diced
- 1/4 cup vegetable broth

- Salt and pepper to taste
- 8 small tortillas (corn or flour)
- Toppings: sliced avocado, diced tomatoes, fresh cilantro, lime wedges

Instructions:

1. Heat the olive oil in a skillet over medium heat.

2. Add the diced onion and minced garlic to the skillet. Sauté for a few minutes until the onion becomes translucent.

3. Add the ground cumin, smoked paprika, and chili powder to the skillet. Stir well to coat the onion and garlic with the spices.

4. Add the cooked black beans and diced sweet potato to the skillet. Pour in the vegetable broth.

5. Season with salt and pepper to taste. Stir everything together.

6. Cover the skillet and simmer for about 10-15 minutes, or until the sweet potato is tender and cooked through.

7. Warm the tortillas in a separate pan or in the oven.

8. Fill each tortilla with the black bean and sweet potato mixture. Top with sliced avocado, diced tomatoes, fresh cilantro, and a squeeze of lime juice.

9. Serve the delicious alkaline black bean and sweet potato tacos as a delightful and nourishing meal.

Nutritional Information:

- Calories: 280
- Carbohydrates: 45g
- Protein: 10g
- Fat: 7g
- Fiber: 10g

Baked Stuffed Bell Peppers with Quinoa and Chickpeas

Description: These colorful bell peppers are filled with a flavorful mixture of quinoa and chickpeas, baked to perfection. They are a nutritious and satisfying meal that is both visually appealing and delicious.

Ingredients:

- 4 large bell peppers (any color)
- 1 cup cooked quinoa
- 1 cup cooked chickpeas
- 1 small onion, diced
- 2 cloves garlic, minced
- 1 teaspoon ground cumin
- 1 teaspoon smoked paprika
- 1/2 teaspoon dried oregano
- Salt and pepper to taste
- 1/4 cup vegetable broth

- Optional toppings: grated cheese, chopped fresh parsley

Instructions:

1. Preheat the oven to 375°F (190°C). Grease a baking dish.

2. Cut the tops off the bell peppers and remove the seeds and membranes from the inside. Set the peppers aside.

3. In a large bowl, combine cooked quinoa, cooked chickpeas, diced onion, minced garlic, ground cumin, smoked paprika, dried oregano, salt, and pepper. Mix well to combine.

4. Spoon the quinoa and chickpea mixture into each bell pepper, filling them to the top. Place the stuffed peppers in the prepared baking dish.

5. Pour the vegetable broth into the bottom of the baking dish.

6. Cover the baking dish with foil and bake for about 30-35 minutes, or until the peppers are tender.

7. Remove the foil and sprinkle grated cheese on top of each stuffed pepper, if desired. Return the peppers to the oven and bake for an additional 5 minutes, or until the cheese is melted and bubbly.

8. Remove the baked stuffed bell peppers from the oven and let them cool for a few minutes.

9. Serve the stuffed bell peppers as a nutritious

and satisfying meal. Garnish with chopped fresh parsley, if desired.

Nutritional Information:

- Calories: 280
- Carbohydrates: 50g
- Protein: 12g
- Fat: 5g
- Fiber: 12g

Weekly Meal Plan Suggestions for Beginners

When embarking on a new journey of healthy eating, planning your weekly meals can be an effective way to stay on track and ensure that you have nutritious and satisfying options available. For beginners, it's important to start with simple recipes that are easy to prepare and incorporate a variety of food groups. In this guide, we will provide you with a sample weekly meal plan that offers a balance of flavors, nutrients, and convenience.

Monday: Breakfast

To kickstart your week, begin with a nutritious and energizing breakfast. Consider starting your day with a bowl of oatmeal topped with fresh berries, nuts, and a drizzle of honey. Oatmeal is a great source of fiber, which aids in digestion and helps keep you full until lunchtime.

Monday: Lunch

For lunch, opt for a colorful and filling salad. Combine a mix of leafy greens, such as spinach and arugula, with roasted vegetables, grilled chicken or tofu, and a tangy vinaigrette dressing. This salad provides a good balance of proteins, healthy fats, and vitamins.

Monday: Dinner

For dinner, try a flavorful and hearty stir-fry. Sauté a variety of colorful vegetables, such as bell peppers, broccoli, and carrots, with your choice of protein, such as shrimp, chicken, or tofu. Season with low-sodium soy sauce and garlic for added flavor. Serve it over a bed of brown rice or quinoa for a complete and satisfying meal.

Tuesday: Breakfast

On Tuesday morning, prepare a delicious and protein-packed smoothie. Blend together frozen berries, a banana, Greek yogurt, and a handful of spinach. This smoothie is not only refreshing but also provides essential nutrients to fuel your day.

Tuesday: Lunch

For a light and refreshing lunch, make a wrap using whole-grain tortillas or lettuce leaves as the base. Fill it with lean turkey or chicken slices, avocado, cucumber, and a sprinkle of feta cheese. This combination offers a good balance of protein, healthy fats, and vegetables.

Tuesday: Dinner

For dinner, try a comforting and nutritious soup. Prepare a vegetable soup using a variety of seasonal vegetables, such as carrots, celery, and zucchini. Add in some cooked lentils or beans for a protein boost. Season it with herbs and spices to enhance the flavor.

Wednesday: Breakfast

On Wednesday morning, enjoy a protein-rich breakfast by

making scrambled eggs with a side of whole-grain toast. Include some sautéed vegetables, such as bell peppers and onions, for added taste and nutrition.

Wednesday: Lunch

For lunch, prepare a nourishing grain bowl. Start with a base of cooked quinoa or brown rice and top it with grilled chicken, roasted vegetables, and a dollop of hummus. This meal provides a good balance of complex carbohydrates, proteins, and healthy fats.

Wednesday: Dinner

For dinner, make a delicious and simple baked salmon. Season the salmon fillets with lemon juice, garlic, and herbs. Bake them in the oven until cooked through. Serve the salmon with steamed asparagus and quinoa for a well-rounded meal.

Thursday: Breakfast

Kickstart your Thursday with a protein-packed breakfast burrito. Fill a whole-grain tortilla with scrambled eggs, black beans, diced tomatoes, and a sprinkle of shredded cheese. Top it with salsa or Greek yogurt for added flavor.

Thursday: Lunch

For lunch, prepare a satisfying and colorful grain salad. Combine cooked farro or barley with roasted vegetables, such as sweet potatoes and Brussels sprouts. Add in some crumbled feta cheese and a drizzle of balsamic vinaigrette. This salad is not only visually appealing but also provides a good mix of carbohydrates, fiber, and vitamins.

Thursday: Dinner

For dinner, try a wholesome and comforting dish like a vegetable stir-fry with tofu. Sauté a medley of vegetables, such as broccoli, bell peppers, and snap peas, in a flavorful sauce made with low-sodium soy sauce, ginger, and garlic. Add in cubes of firm tofu for plant-based protein. Serve it over a bed of brown rice or noodles for a filling and nutritious meal.

Friday: Breakfast

On Friday morning, indulge in a nutritious and tasty breakfast parfait. Layer Greek yogurt, mixed berries, and granola in a glass or jar. This breakfast option is not only delicious but also provides a good balance of protein, fiber, and antioxidants.

Friday: Lunch

For lunch, prepare a satisfying and protein-rich salad. Combine grilled chicken, chickpeas, cucumbers, cherry tomatoes, and feta cheese over a bed of mixed greens. Drizzle it with a light lemon-herb dressing for added flavor. This salad will keep you energized throughout the day.

Friday: Dinner

For dinner, enjoy a delicious and comforting bowl of chili. Use lean ground turkey or beef as the base and add in kidney beans, diced tomatoes, onions, and chili powder. Let it simmer until all the flavors meld together. Serve it with a side of whole-grain bread or brown rice for a filling and satisfying meal.

Saturday: Breakfast

On Saturday morning, treat yourself to a hearty and nutritious breakfast skillet. Sauté a combination of vegetables like bell peppers, onions, and mushrooms with diced sweet potatoes. Add in some cooked turkey sausage or tofu for protein. Top it with a fried or poached egg for an extra boost.

Saturday: Lunch

For lunch, prepare a vibrant and refreshing quinoa salad. Mix cooked quinoa with diced cucumbers, cherry tomatoes, black olives, and crumbled feta cheese. Dress it with a simple lemon-olive oil vinaigrette. This salad is packed with nutrients and is a great option for a light and flavorful midday meal.

Saturday: Dinner

For dinner, try a flavorful and nutritious baked chicken breast with roasted vegetables. Marinate the chicken in a mixture of olive oil, lemon juice, garlic, and herbs. Bake it in the oven until cooked through. Serve it alongside roasted carrots, Brussels sprouts, and sweet potatoes for a well-rounded meal.

Sunday: Breakfast

On Sunday morning, opt for a cozy and filling bowl of overnight oats. Combine rolled oats, almond milk, chia seeds, and your choice of sweetener in a jar. Let it sit in the refrigerator overnight. In the morning, top it with sliced bananas, nuts, and a drizzle of almond butter for a satisfying and nutritious start to the day.

Sunday: Lunch

For a quick and easy lunch, prepare a protein-packed tuna salad. Mix canned tuna with Greek yogurt, diced celery, red onions, and a squeeze of lemon juice. Serve it on whole-grain bread or lettuce leaves for a light and refreshing meal.

Sunday: Dinner

For a comforting and flavorful dinner, make a batch of homemade vegetable curry. Sauté an assortment of vegetables, such as cauliflower, peas, and carrots, in a fragrant curry sauce made with coconut milk and spices. Serve it over brown rice or quinoa for a delicious and nourishing meal.

CHAPTER SIX

Addressing Common

Misconceptions

Debunking Myths and Misconceptions about the Alkaline Diet

The alkaline diet has gained popularity in recent years, with proponents claiming various health benefits. However, there are several myths and misconceptions surrounding this diet that need to be addressed. In this article, we will debunk some of the common misunderstandings about the alkaline diet and provide evidence-based information to help you make an informed decision about your dietary choices.

Myth 1: The Alkaline Diet Can Cure Cancer

One of the most prevalent myths about the alkaline diet is that it can cure cancer. While it is true that cancer cells thrive in an acidic environment, there is no scientific evidence to suggest that following an alkaline diet alone can treat or cure cancer. Cancer is a complex disease that requires proper medical treatment, and relying solely on diet to combat it can be dangerous.

Myth 2: The Alkaline Diet Changes the pH of Your Blood

Another common misconception is that the alkaline diet can significantly alter the pH levels of your blood. The pH level of your blood is tightly regulated by your body's homeostatic mechanisms and does not change significantly based on the foods you eat. While some foods may have a slight impact on the pH levels in your urine, they do not affect the pH of your blood.

Myth 3: All Acidic Foods Are Harmful

Many people mistakenly believe that all acidic foods are harmful to the body. However, it's important to understand that the alkaline diet does not aim to eliminate all acidic foods but rather to promote a balance between acidic and alkaline foods. Our body needs both acidic and alkaline foods to maintain proper functioning. Foods like citrus fruits, tomatoes, and yogurt are acidic in nature but can still be part of a healthy diet.

Myth 4: The Alkaline Diet Promotes Weight Loss

Weight loss is a topic that often comes up in discussions about the alkaline diet. While some proponents claim that an alkaline diet can lead to weight loss, the evidence supporting this claim is limited. It is true that a diet rich in fruits, vegetables, and whole grains can contribute to weight loss, but this is not exclusive to the alkaline diet. Weight loss is more likely attributed to the overall calorie intake and the quality of food consumed rather than the pH level of the diet.

Myth 5: The Alkaline Diet Prevents Osteoporosis

There is a misconception that following an alkaline diet can prevent osteoporosis, a condition characterized by weakened bones. The theory behind this claim is that consuming too many acidic foods can lead to the leaching of calcium from bones, making them weaker. However, scientific studies have not found a significant association between the acidity of the diet and the risk of osteoporosis. Factors such as genetics, hormonal changes, and physical activity play a more significant role in the development of osteoporosis.

Clarifying Misunderstandings and Providing Evidence-Based Information

Now that we have debunked some common myths surrounding the alkaline diet, let's clarify a few misunderstandings and provide evidence-based information about this dietary approach.

The alkaline diet is centered around the concept of maintaining an optimal pH balance in the body. While it is true that certain foods can have an impact on the pH levels in urine, the effects on overall health and disease prevention are not well-established. The human body has a natural buffering system that regulates the pH levels in various organs and tissues, ensuring their proper functioning.

Proponents of the alkaline diet argue that it can promote better digestion, increase energy levels, and improve overall health. However, scientific evidence supporting these claims is limited and inconsistent.

The alkaline diet emphasizes the consumption of alkaline-forming foods such as fruits, vegetables, legumes, and nuts, while discouraging acidic foods like meat, dairy, processed grains, and refined sugars. While it is true that a diet rich in fruits and vegetables can provide essential vitamins, minerals, and antioxidants, it is important to note that the benefits come from the overall nutrient content rather than the pH of the food.

It is crucial to approach the alkaline diet with a balanced perspective. While incorporating more fruits and vegetables into your diet is undoubtedly beneficial, completely eliminating entire food groups, such as dairy or grains, can lead to nutrient deficiencies if not properly planned. It is essential to ensure that you are getting a wide variety of nutrients from different sources to support optimal health.

Moreover, it's worth noting that the human body has its own built-in mechanisms to regulate pH levels. The kidneys and lungs play a vital role in maintaining the acid-base balance in the body, ensuring that the pH levels in our blood and other bodily fluids remain within a narrow range. **The alkaline diet's ability to significantly impact these pH levels is questionable, as the body has robust systems in place to maintain equilibrium.**

When it comes to weight loss, proponents of the alkaline diet argue that acidic foods promote inflammation and weight gain. However, there is no scientific consensus to support this claim. Weight loss is a complex process influenced by various factors, including calorie intake, physical activity, and overall dietary quality. **While the alkaline diet may encourage healthier food choices, it is not a magic solution for weight loss.** Sustainable weight loss requires a balanced diet, portion control, regular exercise, and a comprehensive approach to overall lifestyle habits.

It is important to approach dietary choices based on

evidence-based information rather than relying solely on anecdotal testimonials or expert opinions. While some individuals may report positive experiences with the alkaline diet, it is crucial to remember that individual responses to any diet can vary greatly. **What works for one person may not work for another.**

If you are considering adopting the alkaline diet, it is advisable to consult with a registered dietitian or healthcare professional who can provide personalized guidance based on your specific health needs, goals, and medical history. They can help you design a well-balanced diet that incorporates alkaline-promoting foods while ensuring you meet your nutritional requirements.

Expert Opinions and Testimonials Supporting the Alkaline Diet

While it is important to base dietary decisions on scientific evidence, it is worth mentioning some of the expert opinions and testimonials that support the alkaline diet. It is crucial to note that these opinions are not universally accepted and should be considered alongside scientific research.

Some proponents of the alkaline diet argue that it can improve overall health and well-being by reducing inflammation and promoting a more alkaline state in the body. They suggest that an alkaline environment can support the body's natural detoxification processes, enhance immune function, and even slow down the aging process. However, it is important to remember that these claims are not supported by robust scientific evidence.

It is also worth noting that testimonials from individuals who have followed the alkaline diet often highlight improvements in their energy levels, digestion, and overall well-being. While these personal accounts can be compelling, it is important to recognize that they are subjective experiences and may not be representative of everyone's response to the diet.

Balancing Perspectives and Making Informed Choices

When evaluating the alkaline diet or any other dietary approach, it is essential to consider a balanced perspective that incorporates both scientific evidence and individual experiences. While scientific research forms the foundation of evidence-based recommendations, individual variations, preferences, and lifestyle factors also play a significant role in determining the effectiveness and suitability of a particular diet.

If you are considering the alkaline diet, it is important to approach it with caution and skepticism. **Do thorough research, consult with healthcare professionals or registered dietitians, and critically evaluate the available evidence.** They can provide guidance on how to incorporate alkaline-promoting foods into a well-rounded and nutritionally balanced diet.

Remember that a healthy diet is not solely determined by the pH of the foods we consume. It is about achieving a variety of nutrients, maintaining energy balance, and meeting individual nutritional needs. Prioritize whole foods, including fruits, vegetables, whole grains, lean proteins, and healthy fats, while also ensuring that you consume adequate amounts of essential nutrients.

In summary, debunking myths and misconceptions about the alkaline diet, clarifying misunderstandings with evidence-based information, and considering expert opinions and testimonials help individuals make informed choices about their dietary patterns. While the alkaline diet may have some potential benefits, it is essential to approach it with critical thinking, balance, and an understanding that overall dietary patterns and individual needs are crucial factors in promoting optimal health and well-being.

CHAPTER SEVEN

Overcoming Challenges

and Staying Motivated

Common Challenges Faced When Adopting an Alkaline Diet

The alkaline diet, also known as the acid-alkaline or alkaline ash diet, is based on the idea that certain foods can affect the pH balance of the body. Proponents of this diet claim that consuming alkaline foods can help maintain optimal health and prevent various diseases. However, like any dietary change, adopting an alkaline diet can come with its own set of challenges. In this article, we will explore some common obstacles individuals may face when transitioning to an alkaline lifestyle and discuss strategies to overcome them.

1. Limited Food Choices

One of the primary challenges when adopting an alkaline diet is the limited food choices compared to a standard Western diet. The alkaline diet emphasizes fresh fruits, vegetables, nuts, seeds, and legumes while discouraging acidic foods such as meat, dairy, processed foods, and refined sugars. This shift in dietary habits can be particularly challenging for individuals accustomed to consuming a wide range of acidic foods.

To overcome this challenge, it is essential to focus on the abundance of alkaline foods available. Experiment with new recipes, explore different fruits and vegetables, and get creative with plant-based protein sources like legumes and tofu. Incorporating a variety of flavors, textures, and colors into your meals can make the diet more enjoyable and sustainable. Additionally, it may be helpful to seek inspiration from alkaline recipe books, online resources, and communities to discover innovative ways to prepare alkaline meals.

2. Social Pressures and Dining Out

Another common challenge when following an alkaline diet is dealing with social pressures and dining out. Many social gatherings and restaurants often offer a limited selection of alkaline-friendly options. This can lead to feelings of exclusion or difficulty in maintaining the diet when attending events or dining with friends and family.

To navigate social situations, it is crucial to plan ahead and communicate your dietary preferences to those around you. When invited to a social gathering, offer to bring a dish that aligns with your alkaline diet. This way, you can ensure there is at least one alkaline option available. When dining out, review the menu in advance, and seek out restaurants that offer alkaline-friendly choices. Most restaurants are willing to accommodate special dietary requests if given prior notice. If there are limited options available, focus on selecting the healthiest choices among the available alternatives and make adjustments where possible, such as requesting a salad without acidic dressings.

3. pH Balance Monitoring

Maintaining the desired pH balance within the body is a fundamental aspect of the alkaline diet. However, measuring and monitoring the body's pH levels can be a challenge for individuals new to this approach. Without a clear understanding of their pH levels, it can be difficult to gauge the effectiveness of the diet or identify any necessary adjustments.

To address this challenge, individuals can consider using pH testing strips or pH meters to measure their urine or saliva pH levels. These tools can provide insights into the body's pH balance and help track progress. It is important to note that pH levels can vary throughout the day due to various factors, so it is recommended to measure pH at consistent times, such as in the morning or before meals. Consulting with a healthcare professional or a nutritionist who specializes in the alkaline diet can also provide guidance and support in monitoring pH levels and making necessary adjustments to the diet.

4. Nutritional Adequacy

While the alkaline diet emphasizes whole, nutrient-dense foods, there is a concern that eliminating certain food groups, such as dairy and meat, may lead to potential nutritional deficiencies. Dairy products, for example, are a significant source of calcium, while meat provides essential vitamins and minerals like vitamin B12 and iron.

To ensure nutritional adequacy while following an alkaline diet, it is important to focus on obtaining essential nutrients from alternative sources. For calcium, incorporate calcium-rich plant-based foods like leafy greens, almonds, sesame seeds, and fortified plant-based milk alternatives. Vitamin B12 can be obtained from fortified foods or supplements specifically designed for vegans and vegetarians. Iron can be sourced from legumes, dark leafy greens, seeds, and whole grains. Additionally, consulting with a registered dietitian or nutritionist who specializes in the alkaline diet can help create a well-rounded meal plan that meets all nutritional needs while maintaining the principles of the alkaline diet.

5. Transition Period and Detox Symptoms

When adopting an alkaline diet, some individuals may experience a transition period during which the body adjusts to the new eating patterns. This transition period can sometimes be accompanied by detox symptoms, such as fatigue, headaches, or digestive discomfort. These symptoms can be challenging to manage and may lead to a lack of motivation or a desire to revert to previous dietary habits.

To overcome the challenges of the transition period and detox symptoms, it is essential to be patient with the process. Recognize that these symptoms are temporary and often indicate that the body is undergoing positive changes. Stay hydrated, get adequate rest, and prioritize self-care during this period. Gradually incorporate alkaline foods into your diet, allowing your body to adapt at its own pace. If symptoms persist or become severe, consult with a healthcare professional to ensure proper support and guidance throughout the transition.

Strategies for Overcoming Obstacles and Staying Motivated

Adopting and maintaining a healthy lifestyle requires perseverance and the ability to overcome obstacles that may hinder progress. Whether it's adhering to a new diet, implementing a fitness routine, or making positive lifestyle changes, staying motivated is crucial. In this section, we will explore strategies for overcoming obstacles and maintaining motivation on the path to wellness.

1. Set Clear Goals

Setting clear and realistic goals is essential for staying motivated. Identify what you want to achieve and establish specific, measurable targets. Whether it's losing a certain amount of weight, improving fitness levels, or enhancing overall well-being, clear goals provide focus and direction.

To set effective goals, use the SMART framework: Specific, Measurable, Achievable, Relevant, and Time-bound. For example, instead of setting a goal to "exercise more," specify a goal like "I will exercise for 30 minutes, five days a week, for the next three months." This goal is specific, measurable, achievable, relevant, and time-bound. Writing down your goals and reviewing them regularly will help maintain motivation and track progress.

2. Find Your Why

Understanding your underlying motivations is crucial for sustaining long-term commitment. Take the time to reflect on why you want to make the changes you've set out to achieve. Your "why" can be a powerful source of motivation during challenging times.

Ask yourself questions like: Why is this important to me? How will my life improve by making these changes? What are the long-term benefits I hope to gain? Connecting with your personal reasons and the positive impact these changes will have on your life can fuel your motivation and help you overcome obstacles along the way.

3. Break It Down

Sometimes the journey towards a goal can feel overwhelming, especially if it requires significant lifestyle changes. Breaking your goal into smaller, manageable steps can make the process more approachable and less daunting.

Create an action plan by breaking down your larger goal into smaller, achievable milestones. Each milestone should be specific, measurable, and attainable within a reasonable timeframe. Celebrate your accomplishments along the way to maintain motivation and build momentum. By focusing on one step at a time, you can overcome obstacles and steadily progress towards your ultimate goal.

4. Build a Support System

Having a support system can greatly enhance your motivation and provide accountability. Surround yourself with individuals who share similar goals or who support and encourage your journey towards wellness.

Seek out like-minded individuals by joining fitness groups, online communities, or local classes centered around your specific goals. Engage in discussions, share your progress, and learn from others' experiences. Having a support system can provide valuable guidance, inspiration, and a sense of camaraderie. Additionally, consider sharing your goals with family and friends, who can offer support, understanding, and encouragement throughout your journey.

5. Practice Self-Care

Taking care of your physical and mental well-being is vital for staying motivated and overcoming obstacles. Prioritize self-care activities that nourish and rejuvenate you, such as getting enough sleep, practicing mindfulness or meditation, and engaging in activities you enjoy.

Make self-care a non-negotiable part of your routine. Set aside time each day for activities that promote relaxation, reduce stress, and enhance your overall well-being. When you take care of yourself, you are better equipped to handle challenges, stay motivated, and maintain a positive mindset.

6. Embrace Progress, Not Perfection

Perfection is an unrealistic and often demotivating

expectation. Instead, focus on progress and celebrate even the smallest victories along the way. Acknowledge that setbacks and obstacles are a natural part of the journey and an opportunity for growth.

Recognize and appreciate the progress you make, regardless of how small it may seem. Keep a journal to track your achievements, milestones, and positive changes you've experienced. This reflection can serve as a reminder of how far you've come and boost your motivation to keep going. Remember, it's about progress, not perfection.

CONCLUSION

Recap of the Benefits and Principles of the Alkaline Diet

The alkaline diet, also known as the acid-alkaline diet or alkaline ash diet, is based on the idea that certain foods can affect the pH balance of our bodies. It emphasizes consuming foods that have an alkalizing effect on the body and avoiding those that are acidic. The diet primarily consists of fresh fruits, vegetables, legumes, and whole grains, while limiting the intake of processed foods, refined sugars, and meats. Let's delve deeper into the benefits and principles of the alkaline diet.

One of the primary benefits of the alkaline diet is its potential to promote overall health and well-being. By focusing on nutrient-dense, alkaline foods, this diet can help improve digestion, boost energy levels, and support the immune system. Alkaline foods are typically rich in vitamins, minerals, and antioxidants, which are essential for maintaining a strong and healthy body.

Another advantage of the alkaline diet is its potential to reduce inflammation in the body. Chronic inflammation has been linked to various health conditions, including heart disease, diabetes, and arthritis. By consuming alkaline foods, which have anti-inflammatory properties, individuals may experience a reduction in inflammation and related symptoms.

The alkaline diet is also believed to support healthy weight management. Alkaline foods are generally low in calories and high in fiber, which can help promote satiety and prevent overeating. Additionally, this diet encourages the consumption of fresh fruits and vegetables, which are nutrient-dense and can aid in maintaining a healthy weight.

Furthermore, the alkaline diet promotes the consumption of plant-based foods, which can have a positive impact on the environment. By reducing the intake of animal products and processed foods, individuals following the alkaline diet contribute to lower carbon emissions, conserve water resources, and promote sustainable agricultural practices.

When it comes to the principles of the alkaline diet, there are a few key guidelines to follow. First, it is important to focus on consuming a variety of alkaline foods, such as leafy greens, citrus fruits, berries, nuts, and seeds. These foods have an alkalizing effect on the body and are packed with essential nutrients.

Second, it is recommended to limit the consumption of acidic foods, including processed meats, refined sugars, caffeine, and alcohol. These foods can increase the acidity levels in the body, potentially leading to health issues over time.

Additionally, hydration plays a crucial role in maintaining the alkaline balance in the body. Drinking plenty of water, preferably alkaline or ionized water, can help flush out toxins and maintain proper pH levels.

Lastly, adopting a holistic approach to the alkaline diet is essential. Along with dietary changes, it is important to incorporate regular exercise, stress management techniques, and adequate sleep to support overall health and well-being.

Final Thoughts and Encouragement to Embark on the Alkaline Journey

Embarking on the alkaline journey can be a transformative experience for your health and vitality. By incorporating alkaline foods into your diet and following the principles of the alkaline diet, you can enhance your overall well-being and enjoy the numerous benefits it offers.

It's important to remember that transitioning to an alkaline diet doesn't have to be an all-or-nothing approach. Gradual changes and small steps can lead to long-lasting results. Start by incorporating more alkaline foods into your meals, such as leafy greens, cucumbers, and avocados. Experiment with alkaline recipes and gradually reduce the intake of acidic foods.

As you progress on your alkaline journey, you may start to notice positive changes in your body and overall well-being. Increased energy levels, improved digestion, and a greater sense of vitality are just a few of the benefits that individuals often experience.

Additionally, the alkaline diet can have a positive impact on weight management. By focusing on nutrient-dense, low-calorie foods, you can support healthy weight loss or maintenance. The emphasis on whole grains, fruits, and vegetables provides a wide array of vitamins, minerals, and fiber while keeping you feeling satisfied.

Moreover, the alkaline diet encourages a mindful approach to eating. By being more conscious of the foods you consume, you become more aware of their impact on your body. This can lead to a greater appreciation for fresh, whole foods and a reduction in processed, unhealthy options.

It's important to remember that the alkaline diet is not a cure-all, and individual results may vary. However, many people have reported improvements in various health conditions, such as acid reflux, arthritis, and skin issues, by adopting an alkaline lifestyle.

To stay motivated on your alkaline journey, it can be helpful to set realistic goals and track your progress. Keep a journal of the foods you eat and how they make you feel. This can provide insights into which foods are beneficial for your body and help you make informed choices.

It's also important to seek support and encouragement along the way. Connect with like-minded individuals who are on a similar path or join online communities dedicated to the alkaline lifestyle. Sharing experiences, recipes, and tips can keep you inspired and motivated to stay committed.

Incorporating alkaline habits into your daily routine can be easier with small lifestyle changes. For example, start your day with a glass of warm lemon water to kick-start your digestion and alkalize your body. Replace processed snacks with fresh fruits or raw nuts and seeds. Experiment with alkaline recipes, such as vibrant salads or green smoothies, to add variety and flavor to your meals.

Remember, the alkaline journey is not just about the

physical benefits but also about nourishing your body, mind, and spirit. Prioritize self-care, practice stress management techniques such as meditation or yoga, and get regular exercise to support your overall well-being.

Call-to-Action for Further Resources and Support

If you're ready to embark on the alkaline journey or want to learn more about the alkaline diet, there are several resources and avenues of support available to you. Here are a few options to consider:

1. Books and Literature: Explore books written by experts in the field of alkaline nutrition. Some popular titles include "The Acid-Alkaline Food Guide" by Dr. Susan E. Brown and Larry Trivieri Jr., "The pH Miracle" by Dr. Robert O. Young, and "Alkaline for Life" by Dr. Thomas Barody. These books provide in-depth information, recipes, and practical tips for adopting an alkaline lifestyle.

2. Online Communities and Forums: Join online communities and forums where you can connect with others who are following or interested in the alkaline diet. Websites like Alkaline Diet Exposed and Alkaline for Life offer forums where you can ask questions, share experiences, and find support from like-minded individuals.

3. Professional Guidance: Consider consulting with

a registered dietitian or nutritionist who specializes in alkaline nutrition. They can provide personalized advice, create a tailored meal plan, and address any specific health concerns you may have.

4. Mobile Apps: Explore mobile apps that focus on alkaline nutrition and tracking your alkaline food choices. These apps often provide food lists, recipe ideas, and pH tracking tools to help you stay on track.

Remember, everyone's journey is unique, and it's important to listen to your body and make adjustments that work best for you. While the alkaline diet has its benefits, it's essential to maintain a balanced approach and listen to your body's individual needs.

In conclusion, the alkaline diet offers a range of potential benefits, including improved overall health, reduced inflammation, and support for healthy weight management. By focusing on alkaline foods and following the principles of the diet, you can nourish your body with nutrient-dense foods and promote a more alkaline balance.

Embarking on the alkaline journey requires dedication and a willingness to make changes to your dietary habits. Start by incorporating more alkaline foods into your meals, gradually reducing acidic foods, and paying attention to how your body responds. Small steps can lead to significant improvements in your well-being over time.

Remember to seek support and encouragement from communities, resources, and professionals who specialize in the alkaline diet. They can provide guidance, inspiration, and practical advice to help you stay motivated and make the most of your alkaline journey.

So, if you're ready to experience the potential benefits of the alkaline diet, take that first step today. Embrace the principles, nourish your body with alkaline foods, and embark on a journey toward better health and vitality.

Remember, your alkaline journey is a personal one, and it may take time to fully incorporate the diet into your lifestyle. Be patient with yourself, celebrate your successes, and enjoy the process of discovering new flavors and nourishing your body with alkaline goodness.

Take charge of your health, embrace the alkaline diet, and

witness the positive changes it can bring to your life. Here's to a vibrant and alkaline-filled journey ahead!

Now is the time to take action and start your alkaline journey. Embrace the benefits, principles, and support available to you. Your body will thank you for the nourishment and care it receives from the alkaline diet.

Remember, each step you take toward a more alkaline lifestyle is a step toward optimal health and well-being. Begin today and experience the transformative power of the alkaline diet. Your body, mind, and spirit will thank you for it.